NCLEX
Cardiovascular System 105 Practice Exam Questions

Catherine Black

ISBN-10: 197414464X
ISBN-13: 978-1974144648

Legal Disclaimer

CONTENTS

105 Practice Questions 1.p

Answer Key 110.p

INTRODUCTION

The NCLEX is the examination board that aims to regulate and award nursing qualifications to suitable individuals by way of examination. The NCLEX is only recognized in North American and is needed to practice nursing in USA.

There are two different exams under the NCLEX, that cover the same areas of knowledge. However they aim for different qualifications as well as approach. The exams are NCLEX-RN and NCLEX-PN, RN standing for registered nurse and PN standing for practical nurse.

There are 3 levels of questions, level 1 being the most basic and level 3 being the most advance. The different levels require different levels of thought and knowledge to answer the questions correctly. There is no set number of how many level 1, level 2 or level 3 questions are in the exam. Though the majority will consist of level 2 and 3.

The exams consist of at least 90% of multiple choice questions. Each multiple choice question will have 4options available for the examinee. The questions are mostly scenario based to fit in realistic situations you may face while nursing.

Every individual will experience a different format

of the examination as the exam questions are given one at a time, with the next question dependant on how you answer the previous one. Each person will have a maximum of 6 hours to complete the exam, however there is no minimum time needed. There is a mandatory 10-minute break about 2 ½ hours after the start of the exam and another optional break after about 4 hours of testing.

Your exam is not graded on a bell chart but a pre-existing exam standard. There is also no set requirement on the number of questions to get right to pass. Passing the exam is entirely based on if you have met the required standard of knowledge.

Now that you understand the basic structure of the exam, this book will focus on the cardiovascular system. There are 105 practice questions, all of which are multiple-choice with 4 options available. At the back of the book you will find the answer guide, where the answer and answer explanation is provided.

105 PRACTICE QUESTIONS

Question 1.

You are a nurse caring for a patient who has a recent finding of mitral valve stenosis. You find that the patient is complaining of a cough and breathing difficulty when lying down. The nurse finds a presence of adventitia upon auscultation with tachycardia at a rate of 110 bpm. Which of the following arterial blood gas results should alert the nurse?

- a. PO_2 of 70 mmHg, pCO_2 of 65 mmHg
- b. PO_2 of 88 mmHg, pCO_2 of 40 mmHg
- c. Serum Na of 140 mmol/L (140 mEq/L), HCO_3 of 23 mmol/L (23 mEq/L)
- d. Serum Na of 146 mmol/L (146 mEq/L), HCO_3 of 28 mmol/L (28 mEq/L)

Question 2.

You are a nurse working in emergency who has recently admitted a patient with suspected ventricular fibrillation. You know that in order to appropriately treat this patient, your priority intervention is to:

a. Deliver a synchronized dose of electricity during the QRS cycle
b. Begin CPR at 100bpm
c. Ensure patient is in recovery position
d. Establish IV access in order to administer amiodarone

Question 3.

You are a nurse assessing a patient a few days following open heart surgery. You suspect that the patient has pericarditis. Symptoms of pericarditis include:

    a. Fever and heart failure
    b. Decreased urine output and pedal edema
    c. Crushing chest pain and pedal edema
    d. Leukocytosis and pericardial rub

Question 4.

A patient comes to the chronic disease management clinic after being placed on furosemide the previous week for the treatment of congestive heart failure. The patient reports experiencing muscle spasms, feeling weaker than usual, and having numbness and tingling sensations in extremities. The nurse would expect to recommend the following dietary considerations with the patient:

> a. Increase consumption of carrots and cabbage
> b. Decrease consumption of fish and mushrooms
> c. Increase consumption of bananas and sweet potatoes
> d. Eat watermelon before bed

Question 5.

A patient with a history of an abdominal aortic aneurism (AAA) comes to the emergency room. The nurse should expect that the aneurysm is extending when he complains of:

a. Hypotension and tachycardia
b. Worsening back and abdominal pain
c. Right lower quadrant pain worse with movement and palpation
d. A & B

Question 6.

A patient being discharged from the hospital following open heart surgery, is receiving discharge instructions from the nurse. The patient indicates that teaching is successful when the patient states:

   a. "I need to rub my incisions with a towel thoroughly after showering to prevent infection"

   b. "I need to make sure that I cough often, and walk regularly as soon as I get home."

   c. "I can begin driving my spouse to work tomorrow if I am feeling myself again"

   d. "I should ensure that I am eating three regular sized meals per day when I get home"

Question 7.

A nurse admitting a patient to emergency notes that the patient is presenting with severe chest pain radiating up the jaw. In addition, an electrocardiogram reveals ST-segment elevation in lead II. The nurse expects the physician to order the following laboratory test:

a. BNP
b. Complete blood count (CBC)
c. Troponin level
d. Creatinine kinase

Question 8.

The nurse is providing education to a patient in the chronic disease management clinic who is scheduled to have an inferior vena cava (IVC) filter placed due to a history of pulmonary embolism. This nurse is correct when she explains to the patient that the purpose of an IVC filter is to:

    a.   Prevent a deep vein thrombus from forming in the legs
    b.   Help to dissolve clots before they travel to the lungs in addition to a regimen of anticoagulants
    c.   Prevent clot formation in the lungs
    d.   Trap clots from travelling to the lungs

Question 9.

The nurse is assigned to a patient who has been admitted to the hospital for acute exacerbation of heart failure. The nurse is reviewing the patient's medications during a medication reconciliation. She knows that the following medication will contribute to exacerbation of heart failure in normal doses.

      a. Spironolactone
      b. NSAIDS
      c. Furosemide
      d. Levothyroxine

Question 10.

An unresponsive patient presents to the emergency room with no pulse. The priority of the nurse is to:

a. Establish IV access
b. Acquire a 12 lead ECG
c. Prepare epinephrine
d. Administer oxygen via bag mask

Question 11.

In a patient with insulin dependent diabetes, which clinical presentation would not indicate right-sided heart failure?

a. Peripheral edema
b. Dry cough
c. Jugular venous distention
d. Hepatomegaly

CATHERINE BLACK

Question 12.

A patient brought into the emergency room presents palpitations and dizziness. It is discovered that this patient has the cardiac arrhythmia 'torsades de pointes'. The nurse knows that this means:

a. The patient's ventricles are beating too quickly
b. The patient's atrium are beating faster than the ventricles
c. The patient is having a myocardial infarction
d. The patient is bradycardic

Question 13.

The nurse is performing an electrocardiogram on a patient with a history of atrial fibrillation. The ECG shows an isolated event of a premature ventricular contraction (PVC). At this point, what is the nurse's priority?

a. Immediately notify the physician
b. Prepare the patient for electrical cardioversion
c. Further monitor the patient's ecg/rhythm
d. Prepare to administer intravenous antiarrhythmic medications

Question 14.

A patient female patient scheduled for an angiogram states to the nurse, "I'm not sure that this procedure is right for me." What is the most appropriate way for the nurse to respond to this patient?

a. "Did you read the brochure I gave you?"

b. "How does your husband feel about what you are thinking?"

c. "Don't worry, it's a noninvasive procedure"

d. "Tell me more about why you are feeling this way about the procedure"

Question 15.

The nurse is caring for a patient in the cardiac unit who has been admitted for endocarditis. The patient asks the nurse how someone catches endocarditis. Which of the following would the nurse say is a risk factor for catching endocarditis?

       a. Diabetes
       b. Dental procedures
       c. Diet
       d. Age

Question 16.

A nurse is examining a twelve-lead electrocardiogram tracing taken for a 54-year-old Hispanic male admitted into the Emergency Department following complaints of chest pain and shortness of breath. What would be the expected changes to an ECG wave pattern if the client is suffering from myocardial ischemia?

    a. Raised T waves
    b. A prominent U wave
    c. Wide QRS complex
    d. An inverted U wave

Question 17.

A ward nurse is assigned to care for a client who had cardiac surgery two days ago. What is the most appropriate action for the nurse to take to boost client tolerance for post-operative ambulation?

a. Constantly reassure the client and provide moral support
b. Provide the client with walking aids such as crutches or walkers
c. Administer prescribed analgesics before ambulation
d. Teach the client deep breathing exercises as soon as possible

Question 18.

A 36-year-old female client is complaining of dizziness with vital signs of: pulse rate= 44 beats per minute, blood pressure= 80/60 mm Hg, temperature= 98.3°F. The nurse anticipates which of the following actions?

  a. Preparation of an automated external defibrillator (AED)
  b. Administration of intravenous digoxin
  c. Preparation for transcutaneous external pacing
  d. Ensure hourly monitoring of vital signs

Question 19.

A nurse is reviewing an electrocardiograph strip for an 18-year-old male and sees the following: Heart rate= 84 beats per minute, PR interval= 0.18 second, duration of QRS complex= 0.11 second. The nurse interprets this as:

    a. Normal Sinus Rhythm
    b. Ventricular Fibrillation
    c. First Degree Heart Block
    d. Atrial Fibrillation

Question 20.

A diabetic client on metformin 500 mg twice daily is complaining of recurrent chest pain and is to undergo cardiac catheterization. The nurse knows that the interventions for the procedure should include which of the following?

   a. Metformin is withheld at least 48 hours before the procedure
   b. Metformin dosage is increased 48 hours before the procedure
   c. Metformin dosage is decreased 48 hours after the procedure
   d. Metformin is withheld at least 48 hours after the procedure

Question 21.

A registered nurse is tasked to measure the central venous pressure (CVP) for a newly admitted client to the cardiac care unit. The measured CVP is 6 mm Hg. What is the most appropriate nursing action?

   a. Document the findings
   b. Inform the physician immediately
   c. Initiate a Code Blue
   d. Perform   cardiopulmonary resuscitation (CPR)

Question 22.

A client has recently been diagnosed with hypertension and has been in consultation with the nurse regarding lifestyle changes. Which of the following statements shows an understanding of the necessary dietary restrictions?

a. "I will maintain a diary to record my blood pressure."
b. "I can have salted dried fish for 6 out of 7 days."
c. "I should take my favorite canned beans off the shopping list."
d. "I must take all my medications at the right time every day."

Question 23.

A client is to receive 5.1 mcg of digoxin once daily. The vital signs taken prior to administering the drug are: PR= 54 bpm, BP= 100/70 mm Hg, Temp= 98.5°F. What is the nurse's next action?

    a. Administer the current dose and inform the physician

    b. Withhold the current dose and inform the physician

    c. Administer two times the current dose and inform the physician

    d. Administer half the current dose and inform the physician

Question 24.

A client presenting with the classic symptoms of angina is given sublingual nitroglycerin as an initial treatment. The student nurse observing at the bedside asks the nurse on duty what the tablets are for. Which of the following statements would be the best response?

a. Nitroglycerin is a diuretic that helps the body excrete excess body fluid
b. Nitroglycerin is an antispasmodic that decreases the movement of heart muscles
c. Nitroglycerin is a potent analgesic to reduce chest pain
d. Nitroglycerin is a vasodilator that increases blood flow to the heart

Question 25.

A nurse is caring for a client with deep vein thrombophlebitis who is to be discharged in three days time. It is important for the nurse to emphasize which of the following client teachings?

    a. Legs should be regularly elevated daily for about 10 to 20 minutes every few hours.
    b. Massage the legs with moisturizing lotion on an hourly basis
    c. Aspirin is an appropriate analgesic for pain management
    d. Standing for hours at a time will improve blood circulation

Question 26.

A nurse is assessing a client with peripheral arterial disease. Which of the following signs and symptoms is the most unlikely to be associated with this condition?

    a. Thickened toenails
    b. Discomfort in the client's lower back or buttocks
    c. Grayish blue skin discoloration in the lower extremities
    d. Bounding peripheral pulses

Question 27.

A nurse is conducting a class for clients with permanent pacemakers. Which of the following statements made by a client would indicate an understanding of the health education received?

    a. "I will stay away from the antitheft device at my local store."
    b. "I will use my cellular phone on the opposite side of where I have my pacemaker."
    c. "I have to quit my rugby team."
    d. All of the above

Question 28.

A 35-year-old male client with stable angina is prescribed a nitroglycerin patch by his attending physician. Which of the following statements is an important fact to include with the client's health teaching before discharge?

a. Apply the nitroglycerin patch consistently at the same time each day
b. Contact the emergency medical services immediately upon experiencing dizziness, being lightheaded, and/ or blurring of vision
c. Apply the nitroglycerin patch consistently at the same site each day
d. The nitroglycerin patch should be worn for 24 hours to ensure maximum absorption

Question 29.

A nurse assessing a two-year-old infant, who she suspects has had a cardiac arrest, establishes cardiac function by palpating which artery?

    a. Temporal
    b. Brachial
    c. Carotid
    d. Popliteal

Question 30.

A nurse is caring for a 35-year-old female client who is to receive 5000 units of heparin intravenously as prophylaxis against the formation of deep vein thrombi. She asks the nurse if she can take tablets instead. The nurse is aware that heparin must be given through a parenteral route because:

    a. Heparin irritates the gastric lining therefore causing ulcers
    b. Heparin is absorbed in the small intestine
    c. Heparin is only available as an injection
    d. Heparin is destroyed in the stomach by gastric acids

Question 31.

A nurse is performing a cephalocaudal assessment on a client who is newly diagnosed with hypertension. After auscultating for the apical pulse, the nurse documents a rate of 115 bpm. Which of the following statements about the client is correct?

     a. The client has bradycardia
     b. The client has tachycardia
     c. The client has a normal pulse
     d. The client has tachypnea

Question 32.

The nurse is helping an elderly male client practice Buerger- Allen exercises. The nurse can say that the client has done the exercises in the correct manner if he did which of the following actions?

a. Alternately rotating the foot clockwise and counter clockwise while seated on a chair.
b. Lying flat on the floor while raising the foot up and down
c. Elevating the legs, dangling the legs, and lying flat on the back
d. Alternately raising the right and left foot three inches off the floor while in standing position

Question 33.

A nurse is speaking to a client who is due to have a coronary artery bypass graft (CABG). The client asks the nurse what happens after surgery. Choose the most accurate statement.

a. The client will be on a soft diet immediately after surgery
b. The client will have clear liquids as a first meal after surgery
c. The client will be on a low salt and low fat immediately after surgery
d. The client will be on a high calorie diet for the first 4 days following surgery

Question 34.

A nurse is caring for a patient who has developed cardiac tamponade. What would be an expected nursing action to be included in the client's plan of care?

a. Prepare the patient for a possible chest x-ray
b. Administer fluids orally
c. Place the client in the medical surgical ward
d. Prepare the client for an electrocardiogram (ECG)

Question 35.

A nurse is discussing home care instructions with a 47-year-old male client who is diagnosed with infective endocarditis. The nurse determines that the client has understood the necessary changes to his daily oral hygiene routine when he verbalizes which of the following statements?

    a. "I need to avoid flossing my teeth."
    b. "Oral irrigation devices will help to keep my mouth clean."
    c. "I only need to brush my teeth once a day."
    d. None of the above

Question 36.

An elderly male client tells the outpatient clinic nurse that he is feeling poorly. He is taking various medications to treat both hypertension and cardiac disease. The list of prescribed medications includes digoxin (Lanoxin), spironolactone (Aldactone), and propanolol (Inderal). The attending physician is contemplating an initial diagnosis of digoxin toxicity. Which of the following statements most accurately describes the signs and symptoms of the diagnosis?

- a. Diplopia, decreased libido, difficulty in reading
- b. Tachycardia, nausea, vomiting, impotence, constipation
- c. Double vision, constipation, confusion, increased appetite
- d. Loss of appetite, seeing halos, increased libido

Question 37.

A third-year female student nurse is on her first clinical shift. While observing the various ward activities, she notices a nurse assessing a client who is to undergo cardiac catheterization with the use of a radiopaque dye. The student nurse knows that the most important factor to assess before performing the procedure is:

a. Client allergies to iodine and seafood including shellfish
b. The client's current weight and height
c. The quality of baseline peripheral pulses
d. The client has not eaten any solid food 8 hours prior to the procedure

Question 38.

A 30-year-old Asian female came to the ambulatory clinic for treatment of a persistent pain on her left calf which is swollen and warm to the touch. She regularly takes multivitamins, is on oral contraceptive pills, is fond of leggings and tight jeans, has no family history of cardiac disease, and is an avid hiker. The resident doctor on duty suspects a thrombus formation. Which of the following is the most likely factor that increased the risk of thrombus formation?

a. Being female
b. Use of tight clothing
c. Use of oral contraceptives
d. Being Asian

Question 39.

Enoxaparin (Lovenox) is prescribed to a client as an anticoagulant. The shift nurse is preparing to administer the medication which comes in a prefilled ready-to-use syringe. What is the most appropriate way of administering the drug?

    a. Administer subcutaneously without expelling the air bubble from the syringe

    b. Expel the air bubble from the prefilled syringe and administer on the anterolateral wall of the abdomen

    c. Administer subcutaneously making sure to aspirate first before injection

    d. Expel the air bubble from the prefilled syringe and administer on the posterolateral wall of the abdomen

Question 40.

Balloon valvuloplasty is recommended for an adult female client diagnosed with mitral stenosis. The client asks the nurse if a surgical operation is involved. Which of the following responses is an accurate statement about the procedure?

a. Balloon valvuloplasty is an invasive surgical procedure
b. Balloon valvuloplasty is an invasive nonsurgical procedure
c. Balloon valvuloplasty is a noninvasive surgical procedure
d. Balloon valvuloplasty is a noninvasive nonsurgical procedure

Question 41.

A nurse is formulating a nursing care plan for a client with acute heart failure. The nurse is yet to administer the new physician's order of intravenous dopamine. Which nursing diagnosis is the most appropriate to include in the plan?

a. Increased cardiac output
b. Decreased cardiac output
c. Ineffective cerebral tissue perfusion
d. Risk for activity intolerance

Question 42.

A 57-year-old male client comes to the emergency department complaining of chest pain. He is diagnosed with hypertension and is currently on clonidine (Catapres). The physician makes an initial diagnosis of angina. Which description of pain would support this diagnosis?

- a. Sharp, stabbing pain
- b. Tightening of the chest
- c. Dull, throbbing pain
- d. Intermittent, blooming pain radiating to the neck

Question 43.

An adult male client who is on furosemide (Lasix) has developed hypokalemia. He is then put on another diuretic, spironolactone (Aldactone). Which of the statements should be included as one of the most important points the nurse has to discuss with the client?

a. Avoid using salt substitutes
b. Continue taking the prescribed potassium supplements
c. Sun exposure is part of the treatment
d. Take the medication with meals

Question 44.

A client is rushed to the emergency department due to a hypertensive crisis with a blood pressure of 200/130 mm Hg. The client is experiencing dyspnea, tachycardia, blurred, vision, and confusion. What would be the emergency nurse's first action?

    a. Administer nicardipine (Cardened) intravenously
    b. Keep the client's airway patent
    c. Assess the client's blood pressure every five minutes
    d. Insert a Foley catheter as ordered

Question 45.

A nurse hears a continuous alarm from a cardiac monitor attached to an elderly male client. The client is agitated and distressed over the sound. There are no electrocardiographic complexes on the machine's monitor. What would be the best nursing action?

    a. Help the patient to calm down and check lead placement
    b. Refer the distressed client to a physician
    c. Sedate the client to manage agitation
    d. Call security

Question 46.

The nurse is to administer the first dose of bumetanide (Bumex) IV for a client who was admitted to the unit for congestive heart failure (CHF). The client's vital signs prior to being medicated are: pulse rate of 85 beats per minute, blood pressure of 90/60 mm Hg, respiratory rate of 20 breaths per minute, and oxygen saturation of 98 percent. The client refused to take analgesics for a slight headache with a pain scale rating of 1, stating that: "There is no need for it." Which of the mentioned assessment parameters would be a cause of concern in relation to the prescribed drug?

     a. Pain
     b. Oxygen saturation
     c. Pulse rate
     d. Blood pressure

Question 47.

A client is diagnosed with right-sided heart failure. Which of the following signs and symptoms would the nurse expect to see?

    a. Difficulty in breathing
    b. Jugular vein distention
    c. Crackling lung sounds
    d. Increased appetite

Question 48.

The nurse on duty is utilizing a 6-second strip method to determine the heart rate of a client who has sinus tachycardia. In order to determine the client's ventricular rate for one full minute, which of the following actions would the nurse do?

a. Count the R waves within 5 seconds and multiply the number by 10
b. Count the QRS complexes within 5 seconds and multiply the number by 10
c. Count the R waves within 6 seconds and multiply the number by 10
d. Count the P waves within 6 seconds and multiply the number by 10

Question 49.

A client diagnosed with myocardial infarction is admitted to the coronary care unit. After the morning rounds, the physician orders a transfer to the general ward with instructions to continue cardiac monitoring. Which of the following would the ward nurse allow for the client?

  a. Complete bed rest with bedside commode
  b. Daily ambulation in within 100 feet from the nurse's station
  c. Self-care activities with bathroom privileges
  d. Unrestricted activity and movement

Question 50.

A client is experiencing a bout of ventricular tachycardia. For future similar incidents, the nurse can recommend which of the following client actions?

a. Place a padded spoon between the teeth to avoid injury to the tongue
b. Breathe slowly and steadily through the nose and exhale through the mouth every 3 seconds
c. Loosen restrictive clothing and open the windows
d. Take a big, deep breath and cough out with force every 1-3 seconds

Question 51.

A diabetic and hypertensive client receiving enalapril (Vasotec) is worried about the effects that the medication might have on him. The nurse explains to the client that there are some side effects but it is the adverse effects that he should watch out for. Which of the following is a life threatening adverse effect that the client should immediately report?

    a. Decreased taste sensation
    b. Dry cough
    c. Insomnia
    d. Swelling of the lips

Question 52.

A 57-year-old woman is admitted to the local district hospital for the treatment of peripheral arterial disease. The nurse-in-charge would be most alarmed by which of the following client statements?

a. "I brought my hot water bottle with me from home. Warming my legs before bed helps me to sleep."
b. "I elevate my legs but not too high because it makes me uncomfortable."
c. "I enjoy the exercise program that was recommended to me."
d. "I check my legs everyday to see if anything changed."

Question 53.

A hypertensive 45-year-old male client is having his regular monthly check-up. One of the physician-prescribed medications is lovastatin (Mevacor) which is classified as an antilipemic and is given to decrease the serum levels of cholesterol. Which of the following is an expected side effect of the medication?

    a. Increased levels for liver enzymes
    b. Vomiting, nausea, diarrhea
    c. Tolerable chest pain
    d. Tinnitus

Question 54.

A client is diagnosed with Reynaud's disease. After consultation with the physician, the nurse expects to administer which class of medication?

    a. Vasodilators
    b. Vasoconstrictors
    c. Diuretic
    d. Antilipemics

Question 55.

An elderly female client is diagnosed with myocarditis. She asks the nurse about the prognosis of her condition. The best nursing response would be:

a. Cardiac surgery needs to be performed to accomplish full recovery
b. The condition resolves on its own without a specific treatment
c. Anticoagulant therapy will greatly improve the condition
d. A sedentary lifestyle will be necessary

Question 56.

The nurse is teaching a client, non-pharmacologic interventions, to help boost response to pain medication prescribed for angina. Which of the following, if verbalized by the patient, would indicate a correct understanding of the health teaching?

    a. "I will limit my weekly alcohol intake to two beers only."

    b. "I will join a meditation class to help me relax."

    c. "I will stop smoking immediately."

    d. "I will do thirty minutes of aerobic exercise daily."

Question 57.

The nurse is evaluating the laboratory results for a client with myocardial infection. Which of the following laboratory values would support the client's diagnosis?

- a. Elevated hematocrit
- b. Raised creatinine phosphokinase (CPK)
- c. Elevated white blood cell (WBC) count
- d. Raised serum ferretin

Question 58.

A middle-aged, male, asthmatic client is diagnosed with hypertension and is to receive sotalol (Betapace) to manage his elevated blood pressure. Which of the following nursing interventions is the priority for this situation?

    a. Consider discussing the change of medication with the physician
    b. Administer the medication as ordered orally
    c. Assess the patient's blood pressure
    d. Assess the patient's pulse

Question 59.

A client is to undergo a coronary artery bypass grafting procedure. The nurse is preparing to conduct a health education session for the client. Which of the following would be an accurate statement to include in the health teaching?

a. The client will be placed on a mechanical ventilator
b. A radiopaque dye will be used
c. The client should continue taking his medications until right before the procedure
d. A balloon-tipped catheter will be inserted

Question 60.

Gemifibrozil is an antilipemic medication prescribed to a male client. The nurse advises the client to inform the physician of any other medication he might be taking. Which medication classification should the physician be aware of?

    a. Anticoagulants
    b. Analgesics
    c. Diuretics
    d. Vasodilators

Question 61.

A coronary care unit nurse is examining an electrocardiograph strip for one of the clients admitted to the unit. The nurse notes that there are premature ventricular contractions every other heart beat. The nurse documents this finding as:

      a. Couplet
      b. Quadrigeminy
      c. Trigeminy
      d. Bigeminy

Question 62.

A client who has developed cardiac tamponade is scheduled for pericardiocentesis. Which postoperative assessment parameter would indicate an unsuccessful treatment?

    a. Elevated central venous pressure (CVP)
    b. Elevated blood pressure
    c. Clearly audible heart sounds
    d. Client verbalizes relief

Question 63.

Part of the diagnostic interventions ordered for a client is a magnetic resonance imaging of the heart. The nurse should alert the medical team immediately if the client has which of the following?

    a. An allergy to shellfish and iodine
    b. A permanent pacemaker
    c. A medical diagnosis of insulin dependent diabetes mellitus
    d. A nasogastric tube

Question 64.

The physician is performing cardioversion on a client suffering from supraventricular tachydysrhythmia. Which of the following would be a cause of concern during the procedure?

    a. The client is on continuous oxygen at 4Lpm via nasal cannula

    b. All the medical personnel present stays away from the client's bed when the countershock is being delivered

    c. The skin of the client's chest is dry

    d. The client's jewelry and watch are removed

Question 65.

The physician orders dobutamine for a client currently undergoing a cardiopulmonary bypass surgery. The nurse knows that the side effects for adrenergic agonists include which of the following?

   a. Urinary urgency
   b. Angina
   c. All of the above
   d. None of the above

Question 66.

A client is complaining of severe chest tightness that happens at approximately the same time daily even when in bed. The client does not think there are any factors that cause the onset of chest tightening. Which type of angina would the nurse suspect?

    a. Prinzmetal's angina
    b. Stable angina
    c. Unstable angina
    d. Chronic angina

Question 67.

A client with cardiac dysrhythmia received an intravenous dose of procainamide (Procanbid) as treatment. Soon after the administration, the client verbalizes feelings of dizziness. What would be the best nursing intervention?

    a. Let the client lie flat on his back until the dizziness stops

    b. Assess the client's apical pulse and blood pressure

    c. Connect the patient to a cardiac monitor

    d. Apply a nitroglycerin patch

Question 68.

A community based nurse is scheduled to make a home visit for an elderly female client whose neighbor recently had sclerotherapy. The client asks the nurse about the procedure as she has varicose veins on both her lower limbs. The most accurate answer would be:

    a. The varicose veins are manually removed through surgery

    b. A fluid is injected into the vein that causes it to close

    c. The vein is tied off at one end and removed

    d. Oral medication is taken for six months that causes the varicose veins to close

Question 69.

A client has just undergone surgery for the placement of a vena caval filter. As part of the postoperative interventions for this type of surgery, the nurse puts the client in which position?

    a. Sitting with the back at a 45-degree angle
    b. Lying flat on the back
    c. Sitting with the back at a 90-degree angle
    d. Lying flat on the stomach

Question 70.

The nurse is monitoring the digoxin serum levels of an elderly client. A client with digoxin toxicity would most likely have which laboratory value?

    a. 3.0 ng/mg
    b. 2.0 ng/mg
    c. 1.0 ng/mg
    d. 0.5 ng/mg

Question 71.

An elderly female client comes to the emergency department with several complaints that include: difficulty of breathing without physical exertion, swelling on both legs, feeling tired and weak, and gaining weight. The nurse is most likely to suspect that the client has which condition?

    a. Endocarditis
    b. Heart Failure
    c. Bronchial Asthma
    d. Myocarditis

Question 72.

A client with stable angina is prescribed with nitroglycerin tablets to be taken sublingually. The nurse is teaching the client about the correct drug usage when angina episodes occur. Which of the following is the best instruction?

a. Have one tablet every fifteen minutes until the episode passes

b. Have one tablet initially, two tablets after five minutes, and call the physician if the pain is not relieved after taking a total of 3 tablets

c. Have one tablet initially, one tablet after five minutes, one tablet after another five minutes, and call the physician if the pain is not relieved after taking a total of 3 tablets

d. Have one tablet every fifteen minutes and call the physician

Question 73.

Prior to administering the prescribed digoxin, the nurse checks the client's apical pulse. The nurse accurately performs the procedure if auscultation is done at which landmark?

a. Left midclavicular line at the fourth intercostal space
b. Right midclavicular line at the fourth intercostal space
c. Left midaxillary line at the second intercostal space
d. Right midaxillary line at the second intercostals space

Question 74.

A community nurse is conducting a health education seminar about the diet restrictions for hypertensive clients. The clients are suggested to make lists of food that they think have a low sodium content. Which of the following item would have the lowest sodium level?

      a. Demineralized water
      b. Cough syrup
      c. Sleeping pills
      d. Toothpaste

Question 75.

Before administering the prescribed lidocaine dose to a client, the nurse carefully checks the label on the vial. This check is necessary to identify which of the following?

    a. The manufacturing date
    b. The additives or components
    c. The brand name
    d. The color of the drug

Question 76.

A male client is receiving an infusion of streptokinase (Stratptas) when he suddenly presents with difficulty of breathing, severe anxiety, and generalized itchiness. The nurse caring for the client identifies stridor upon auscultation and lowered blood pressure after further assessment. What is the is most critical nursing action?

a. Put the client on 4Lpm of oxygen via nasal cannula
b. Slow down the infusion and assist the client to a semi-Fowler's position
c. Administer an antihistamine before continuing the infusion
d. Stop the infusion and inform the physician

Question 77.

A client was found to have and abdominal aortic aneurysm. The client expresses a reluctance to comply with the lifestyle changes needed to reach the goal of treatment. The nurse's best response would be which of the following?

    a. "Some lifestyle changes are necessary to keep the disease from progressing"

    b. "Lifestyle changes are important to help completely cure the disease"

    c. "Minor changes will greatly contribute to stopping the disease"

    d. "Lifestyle changes are not as important as medication"

Question 78.

Isosorbide dinitrate (Isordil Titradose) is prescribed for a client to manage anginal pain. The client complains of headache, having dry mouth, and sudden dizziness and weakness when standing up from a seated position. What would be the best action for the attending nurse to take?

a. Document the client's complaints and inform the physician immediately
b. Document the client's complaints and withhold the medication
c. Document the client's complaints and reeducate the client on the drug's side effects
d. Document the client's complaints and reduce the drug dosage

Question 79.

Nicotinic acid is prescribed for a client as treatment for hyperlipidemia. Which of the following statements would indicate effective health education by the nurse?

    a. "I do not need to stop drinking alcoholic beverages."
    b. "I need to take my medication thirty minutes before meals."
    c. "I should expect tarry-colored stool as an expected effect of the medicine."
    d. "I can take aspirin thirty minutes before taking nicotinic acid to help avoid flushing."

Question 80.

A middle-aged female client is diagnosed with stable angina. The nurse is helping the client identify situations that may trigger an anginal episode. The client shows an understanding of the discussion if she verbalizes which of the following statements?

    a. "I will increase my water intake to avoid constipation"

    b. "I need to constantly wear a jacket even when it is sunny"

    c. "Weight lifting is a good way to stay fit"

    d. "I can eat big heavy meals three times in a day"

Question 81.

On the second hour of the morning shift, a ward nurse is reviewing the medication records of four new admissions. All clients are on hypertensive medications. Which client would be at the highest risk for hypokalemia?

a. Client prescribed with spironolactone (Aldactone)
b. Client prescribed with furosemide (Lasix)
c. Client prescribed with triamterene (Dyrenium)
d. Client prescribed with amiloride (Midamor)

Question 82.

A 56-year-old male client complaining of chest tightening is found to have myocardial infarction. To determine the location of damage to the myocardium, which diagnostic tool is most likely to be used?

    a. Electrocardiogram (ECG)
    b. Blood work up (Cardiac Enzymes)
    c. Auscultation of the apical pulse
    d. Cardiac catheterization

Question 83.

While performing daily rounds, a ward nurse witnesses a male client collapse while ambulating. The client has a family history of heart disease. What is the best initial nursing intervention?

    a. Refer the client to a physician
    b. Assess the client
    c. Perform CPR
    d. Move the client to a bed

Question 84.

A 47-year-old female client is diagnosed with atrioventricular heart block. She heard her attending physician mention "Mobitz II" and asks the nurse what it all means. The most accurate answer would be which of the following statements?

    a. Mobitz II is another name for a third-degree atrioventricular heart block

    b. Mobitz II is another name for an atrioventricular heart block II

    c. Mobitz II is another name for a second-degree atrioventricular heart block

    d. Mobitz II is another name for a complete heart block

Question 85.

The nurse is performing a 12-lead ECG for a client with angina. The tracing shown on the machine's monitor is a continuous up and down erratic wave with no specific pattern. What is the nurse's next course of action?

    a. Initiate cardiopulmonary resuscitation (CPR)
    b. Check the lead placement
    c. Shave the client's whole chest
    d. Inform the physician

Question 86.

Heparin is prescribed for a client with deep vein thrombosis. In case of bleeding and hemorrhage, the nurse should keep which drug on hand?

    a. Vitamin K
    b. Vitamin C
    c. Protamine Sulfate
    d. Protamine Citrate

Question 87.

A 75-year-old female client is admitted into the accident and emergency department with complaints of severe chest pain and numbness in the left shoulder and arm. The physician identifies the diagnosis as acute myocardial infarction (MI). STAT orders include: a 12-lead ECG, chest x-ray, oxygenation via nasal cannula at 4 liters per minute, cardiac profile, morphine 3 mg IV. What would be the nurse's first action?

   a. Administer morphine intravenously
   b. Obtain an electrocardiograph reading
   c. Collect specimens for required diagnostics
   d. Send the patient to the radiology department for a chest x-ray

Question 88.

A nurse working at an outpatient facility is caring for a 46-year-old male client with complaints of a runny nose and dry cough. While the respiratory rate is being taken, he clutches his chest and says he is in pain. Which of the following queries would be most helpful in identifying pain that is not cardiac in origin?

- a. "On a scale of 1 to 10, with 1 being the lowest score and 10 being the highest, how would you rate your pain?"
- b. "Is this pain a new occurrence?"
- c. "How would you describe the pain you are feeling?"
- d. "Does the chest pain worsen when you take a breath?"

Question 89.

A 54-year-old male client is prescribed with a loop diuretic as one of the medications to manage hypertension. Which of the following drug names would the nurse expect to administer?

a. Urea (Ureaphil)
b. Ethacrynic Acid (Edecrin)
c. Methazolamide
d. Amiloride

Question 90.

A student nurse on clinical rotation is tasked by the instructor to check a client's blood pressure. The instructor identifies that the student nurse has correctly done the procedure when which of the following situations is avoided?

    a. The client is seated comfortably and the blood pressure is measured on an arm that is supported and raised to the level of the heart

    b. Taking the client's blood pressure after being rested for fifteen minutes after smoking

    c. Using the appropriate blood pressure cuff for the arm circumference of the client

    d. Taking the client's blood pressure with a newly calibrated sphygmomanometer

Question 91.

A client is experiencing supraventricular tachydhysrhythmia. The physician is contemplating on utilizing vagal maneuvers as treatment and the nurse is instructed to prepare for a carotid sinus massage. Which of the following preparatory actions is appropriate?

    a. Keep a crash cart, defibrillator, and other resuscitative implements within easy reach
    b. Instruct the client to void and empty the bladder
    c. Collect necessary specimens for blood testing
    d. Instruct the client to keep the head facing straight ahead

Question 92.

An unconscious, elderly, male client was brought to the emergency room by his two adult children. After assessment and initial treatment to stabilize the client, the physician's diagnosis is myocardial infarction. The information is relayed to the client's children using the layman's term which is:

    a. Brain attack
    b. Heart attack
    c. Stroke
    d. Syncope

Question 93.

A client with a history of peptic ulcer disease is admitted to the emergency care unit with a chief complaint of severe chest pain. The nurse is aware that the general treatment for chest pain is morphine, oxygenation, nitrates, and aspirin. Which of the mentioned treatments, if ordered by a physician, would be a possible cause for concern?

    a. Morphine
    b. Oxygen
    c. Nitrates
    d. Aspirin

Question 94.

A client is scheduled for digital subtraction angiography. Prior to the procedure, the nurse identifies that the client has an allergy to iodine. What would be the appropriate nursing intervention?

    a. Cancel the appointment
    b. Obtain a physician's order for antihistamines
    c. Reschedule the appointment after two weeks
    d. Continue with the procedure

Question 95.

A client has undergone vein stripping and ligation as treatment for unsightly varicose veins on the left leg. The client has hypersensitivity on the affected limb. What is the best nursing intervention after client assessment?

   a. Refer the client to a physician
   b. Elevate the client's left leg
   c. Apply a warm compress to the affected site
   d. Administer analgesics

Question 96.

A client has been found to have ventricular fibrillation. The physician defibrillates the client at 200 Joules. After the first shock, the nurse prepares the machine settings for the next defibrillation. At what therapeutic level should the energy be set?

      a. 500 Joules
      b. 400 Joules
      c. 300 Joules
      d. 200 Joules

Question 97.

A nurse is observing a client who is consistently experiencing episodes of ventricular tachycardia. What makes this condition life-threatening?

    a. Ventricular tachycardia can cause myocardial ischemia
    b. Ventricular tachycardia cannot be treated with through defibrillation
    c. Ventricular tachycardia is irreversible
    d. Ventricular tachycardia is a frightening experience for the client

Question 98.

A client was admitted a week ago with a final diagnosis of thrombophlebitis. While eating breakfast the client becomes agitated, breathless, and is complaining of chest pain. The nurse assesses the client for which condition?

    a. Myocardial infarction
    b. Pulmonary embolism
    c. Unstable angina
    d. Heartburn

Question 99.

A temporary pacemaker is inserted on the left subclavian vein of a client being cared for at a surgery ward. To avoid complications, the nurse is expected to carry out which of the following interventions?

a. Providing the client with a walker to use while ambulating
b. Massaging the client's left arm
c. Avoiding sudden movements to the left arm
d. Massaging the client's right arm

Question 100.

A patient at the intensive care unit has gone into asystole. After calling for help and initiating a code blue, the nurse's next action would be which of the following?

    a. Perform cardiopulmonary resuscitation
    b. Start defibrillation
    c. Obtain a 12-lead ECG
    d. Administer lidocaine intravenously as ordered

Question 101.

A ward nurse mentoring a nursing student is discussing the helpful information a client needs to know when wearing a Holter monitor. The student demonstrates correct understanding of the discussion with which statement?

    a. The client should avoid bathing in showers and bathtubs
    b. The client needs to limit physical activity and movement
    c. The client wears the Holter monitor for 12 hours
    d. The client should take off the Holter monitor before bed

Question 102.

An echocardiogram is ordered for a client with shortness of breath to rule out cardiac disease as a cause of dyspnea. Which of the following statements about an echocardiogram is false?

    a. It is a noninvasive procedure
    b. It is similar to an ultrasound
    c. It is an invasive procedure
    d. It involves putting the client in a supine position

Question 103.

A client is to undergo valve replacement. When in consultation with the members of the healthcare team, the client shows confusion about the different types of valve options. Which of the following choices are classified as bioprosthetic valves?

   a. Bovine valves
   b. Mechanical prosthetic valves
   c. Canine valves
   d. Feline valves

Question 104.

A client with acute myocardial infarction and a history of stroke and deep vein thrombosis is prescribed with thrombolytic medications. Ten units of reteplase (Retavase) IV bolus is ordered by the physician. What would be the nurse's possible reason for refusing to administer the medication?

    a. The client has a history of stroke
    b. The client has a history of DVT
    c. The drug dosage is too high
    d. The drug dosage is too low

Question 105.

A client has developed Dressler's syndrome during a two-month stay at the hospital. The nurse shows an understanding of the condition with which of the following statements?

a. Dressler's syndrome is a nosocomial disease
b. Dressler's syndrome is a community-acquired disease
c. Dressler's syndrome is complication of myocardial infarction
d. Dressler's syndrome is a complication of pericarditis

105 ANSWER KEY

1.

Answer- A

Explanation: A diagnosis of mitral valve stenosis complications (heart failure) is evidenced by an increase in PCO2 levels and decreased in PO2 levels. Some common signs of heart failure in individuals with mitral valve stenosis are:

-Jugular venous distention
-Cold clammy skin
-Tachycardia
-Increased pCO2
-Decreased pO2

The other lab values are normal.

2.

Answer- B

Explanation: Using priorities of intervention (airway, breathing, circulation), the correct answer is B, as it is important to re-establish proper circulation immediately; the pads are placed on the patient during CPR. IV access is to be initiated at a later time following the initiation of CPR.

Answer C is not correct, as placing a patient in the recovery position does not allow the nurse to re-establish circulation and impedes CPR.

3.

Answer- D

Explanation: Patients with pericarditis often present with fever, leukocytosis, pericardial rub, and crushing chest pain. Edema and heart failure can be complications of pericarditis; however, they are not direct symptoms of pericarditis.

4.

Answer- C

Explanation: This patient is likely experiencing decreased serum potassium levels. Furosemide is potassium wasting diuretic, meaning that more than the usual amount of potassium is wasted in the urine. Bananas and sweet potatoes are two foods known to be high in potassium. This patient will likely also need to have his/her electrolyte levels drawn, as altered potassium levels can be detrimental to normal cardiac functioning.

5.

Answer- D

Explanation: Common symptoms of AAA include

hypotension, tachycardia, and back and abdominal pain. Right lower quadrant pain is more consistent with appendicitis. Worsening back and abdominal pain may indicate that the aneurysm is beginning to push on the lumbar nerves.

6.

Answer- B

Explanation: Deep breathing, activity, and coughing lowers the risk of pulmonary embolisms, blood clots, and pneumonia. Driving following open heart surgery should be at the advice of a physician, and the operation of machinery is not advised following open heart surgery. It is important to eat small frequent meals throughout the day following surgery, and slow progression to a regular diet can be made after time. Rubbing incisions can lead to irritation and infection, and dehiscence of wounds. It is important to pat the incision sites dry gently.

7.

Answer- C

Explanation: The diagnostic test for myocardial infarction is a Troponin level.

8.

Answer- D

Explanation: An IVC filter is used to prevent emboli from travelling from the extremities (primarily the legs) to the lungs, and becoming trapped in the pulmonary capillary network. The filter is not designed to prevent clot formation, or dissolve clots.

9.

Answer- B

Explanation: NSAIDS or nonsteroidal anti-inflammatory drugs are known to cause fluid and sodium retention, a major contributing factor to exacerbation of heart failure and fluid overload. Although levothyroxine in high doses can lead to an exacerbation of heart failure, a normal regimen will not. It is important for a patient to continue taking the prescribed dose of levothyroxine in order to ensure normal thyroid functioning. Spironolactone and Furosemide are both diuretics that are used in the treatment of heart failure.

10.

Answer- D

Explanation: Although the priority is to begin CPR, it is important to maintain a flow of oxygen that will be circulated during CPR. Although correct, the other options are not a priority in a patient presenting as pulseless and unresponsive.

11.

Answer- B

Explanation: The information regarding insulin dependent diabetes is placed to throw off the reader, and is typical of the NCLEX examination. Patients with right sided heart failure will have systemic blood backup into the vena cava. This will result in edema, jugular vein distension, and hepatomegaly. Although a symptom of some medication used to treat heart failure, dry cough is not a symptom of right-sided heart failure.

12.

Answer- A

Explanation: Torsade de pointe (twisting of the point) refers to a formation on the electrocardiogram that looks like a wave. This means that the patient is experiencing ventricular tachycardia. Although a myocardial infarction may be a precipitating factor, the nurse, at this point, does not know this information. The patient cannot be bradycardic if they are experiencing ventricular tachycardia.

13.

Answer- C

Explanation: An isolated event of a premature ventricular contraction is not a life-threatening condition. If it continues, it may develop into something more serious, however,the appropriate intervention is for the nurse to continue monitoring the patient. It is not necessary for the nurse to notify the physician, as this is not immediately life threatening.

14.

Answer- D

Explanation: The most appropriate response is for the nurse to engage the patient in therapeutic conversation. The other answers do not seek to address the direct concerns that the patient may have.

15.

Answer- B

Explanation: Major risk factors for developing endocarditis include the following:
- Mechanical heart valve replacement
- Dental Procedures
- IV Drug Use
- Immunosuppression

16.

Answer- D

Explanation: One of the hallmark electrocardiographic changes caused by myocardial ischemia is an inverted or negative U wave.

Raised and tall T waves are indicative of hyperkalemia.

A prominent U wave is seen in patients with bradycardia and those with severe hypokalemia.

A widened QRS complex is seen in bundle branch blocks and other conditions that cause delays to the heart's intraventricular conduction.

17.

Answer- C

Explanation: For the initial forty-eight to seventy-two hours post cardiac surgery, it is most appropriate for the nurse to promote the use of analgesics to address pain management. This allows for more client participation in other post operative activities such as walking and deep breathing.

All the other options are not helpful in encouraging the client to ambulate.

18.

Answer- C

Explanation: Dizziness and low blood pressure are two indications of a decrease in the cardiac output. Transcutaneous pacing is a temporary measure to help remedy this.

Defibrillation and vital signs monitoring are an immediate priority while digoxin will further lower down the pulse rate.

19.

Answer- A

Explanation: The characteristics of a normal sinus rhythm are:
- Heart rate of 60-100 beats per minute
- QRS duration of < 0.12 second
- PR interval of 0.12- 0.20 second

20.

Answer- A

Explanation: Metformin is withheld 48 hours before cardiac catheterization to eliminate the risk of lactic acidosis usually related to the iodine dye used.

21.

Answer- A

Explanation: The normal range for central venous pressure (CVP) is from 3 to 8 mm Hg.

22.

Answer- C

Explanation: The recommended dietary restrictions for a hypertensive client include cholesterol and sodium such as table salt and MSG (monosodium glutamate). Avoiding canned food is appropriate while having dried salted fish regularly is not.

The other options are not related to dietary restrictions.

23.

Answer- B

Explanation: Digoxin can cause bradycardia and it is important to check the apical pulse before administration. It is best to withhold the drug for clients with pulse rates of below 60 bpm and refer to a physician before proceeding with further treatment.

24.

Answer- D

Explanation: Nitroglycerin's mechanism of action involves reducing the oxygen demand and consumption of the heart's myocardium through peripheral vasodilation.

25.

Answer- A

Explanation: Elevating the lower extremities, ideally above the level of the heart, promotes venous return and reduces stasis. Other client teachings include:
-inspecting the lower extremities for signs of edema and accurately measuring leg circumference
- wearing thigh or knee high antiembolism stockings
-recognizing the signs and symptoms of bleeding
-be aware of the dangers associated with anticoagulant medications
-avoidance of restrictive and constricting clothing

The other options are contraindicated for this condition.
26.

Answer- D

Explanation: Clients with peripheral arterial disease are more likely to exhibit decreased or even absent peripheral pulses.

The other options are characteristic assessment findings

of the mentioned disease.

27.

Answer- D

Explanation: All of the statements are correct. Health education for clients with pacemakers includes:
- Staying away from antitheft devices and transmitter towers
- Keeping cellular phones away from the pacemaker
- Avoid rough activities which includes contact sports

28.

Answer- A

Explanation: Applying the nitroglycerin patch at a regular time will ensure that the body has the therapeutic amount of the medication.

Dizziness, lightheadedness, and blurring of vision are normal side effects of wearing a nitroglycerin patch. Rotating the patch sites daily is recommended to avoid skin irritation. The patch is generally worn over a 12- to 14-hour time span to allow for nitrate free periods that help to prevent drug dependence and tolerance.

29.

Answer- B

Explanation: For infants, the brachial pulse is palpated at the crook of the elbow.

30.

Answer- D

Explanation: Heparin is administered intravenously or subcutaneously as it is easily destroyed by gastric secretions in the stomach.

31.

Answer- B

Explanation: The normal pulse or heart rate for an adult is 60-100 beats per minute. Tachycardia is defined as having more than 100 beats per minute.

Bradycardia is having a pulse less than 60 beats per minute while tachypnea refers to having more than 20 breaths per minute.

32.

Answer- C

Explanation: Buerger- Allen exercises are done through three steps. The first step is elevating the feet until blanching occurs and the second one is dangling them until the skin reddens. Thirdly the client lies stretched out and flat on the back. Steps are done for approximately three minutes each. The purpose is to promote arterial circulation throughout the lower extremities most especially to the feet.

33.

Answer- B

Explanation: Initially the client will be put on clear liquids postoperatively but will eventually progress to a diet that is low in fat and salt.

34.

Answer- A

Explanation: The diagnostics for a client who has developed cardiac tamponade include a chest x-ray or an echocardiogram. It is recommended to administer fluids intravenously as treatment for a lowered cardiac output. Placing the client in a critical care unit is likewise important for monitoring of hemodynamics.

35.

Answer- A

Explanation: It is important to stress the avoidance of

flossing and the use of oral irrigation devices that could cause bacteremia. Oral hygiene should be performed at least two times daily with a soft toothbrush.

36.

Answer- A

Explanation: Some of the early signs that point to digoxin toxicity are having double vision or diplopia, nausea, and decreased appetite or anorexia. Other signs and symptoms of toxicity are confusion, decreased libido, impotence, and visual disturbances, and gastrointestinal problems such as:

- Seeing spots and/ or halos
- Photophobia
- Green or yellow vision
- Vomiting
- Diarrhea

37.

Answer- A

Explanation: All the options are appropriate for preprocedural assessment however the most critical factor to assess is client allergy to seafood and iodine as the radiopaque dye may cause an anaphylactic reaction.

38.

Answer- C

Explanation: The use of oral contraceptive pills (OCP) is one of the contributory risk factors of thrombus formation. Other risk factors include:

- Venous stasis possibly caused by immobility, varicose veins, or heart failure
- Disorders affecting blood coagulation
- Pregnancy
- Pelvic injuries
- Fracture of the lower extremities
- Venous injuries caused by frequent intravenous injections of irritants as in chemotherapy

39.

Answer- A

Explanation: Enoxaparin (Lovenox) is only administered through subcutaneous injection to either the anterolateral or posterolateral wall of the client's abdomen. There is no need for aspiration when injecting. Expelling the air bubble on the prefilled medication syringe is likewise not recommended.

40.

Answer- B

Explanation: Balloon valvuloplasty for mitral stenosis is an invasive but nonsurgical procedure that involves placing a balloon catheter through the atrial septum all the way to the mitral valve to improve blood circulation and cardiac output.

41.

Answer- B

Explanation: Clients with heart failure have a decreased cardiac output. Dopamine is prescribed to increase the contractility of the myocardium which in turn increases the cardiac output and improves blood flow to the kidneys and the periphery. This promotes fluid excretion that improves fluid retention and edema.

42.

Answer- B.

Explanation: The pain experienced by clients with angina is most often described as squeezing, tightening, burning, and like having a weight or pressure on the chest.

43.

Answer- A

Explanation: Spironolactone is a potassium-sparing diuretic that promotes retention of potassium. It is imperative to caution the client against eating potassium-rich food including salt substitutes. Exposure to direct sunlight should also be avoided.

44.

Answer- B

Explanation: In an emergency, the priority is to maintain a patent airway. All the other interventions are appropriate but not the foremost action.

45.

Answer- A

Explanation: The client's distress and agitation stems from the sounds made by the cardiac monitor's alarm. The most appropriate way to handle the situation is to resolve the specific issue that is causing the alarm.

46.

Answer- D

Explanation: Bumetanide is a diuretic that can potentially cause lowered blood pressure as a side effect.

All the other vital signs are within normal range and the pain experienced by the client is tolerable.

47.

Answer- B

Explanation: The signs and symptoms of right-sided heart failure are usually related to the systemic circulation while those for left-sided heart failure are evidenced by disturbances to the pulmonary system.

48.

Answer- C

Explanation: To determine the ventricular rate for one full minute, the number of R waves or QRS complexes is counted within 6 seconds. The value is then multiplied by 10.

49.

Answer- C

Explanation: The most appropriate allowance for a newly transferred patient from the coronary care unit is to have bathroom privileges and to do self care. Ambulation is also recommended with supervision and to be progressively increased over time.

50.

Answer- D

Explanation: One of the client recommendations for those with unstable ventricular tachycardia is to perform self cardiopulmonary resuscitation through coughing, otherwise known as cough CPR.

51.

Answer- D

Explanation: A potentially life threatening adverse effect of enalapril is angioedema. Swollen lips can cause an airway obstruction that could endanger the client. All the other options are expected side effects of the medication.

52.

Answer- A

Explanation: Peripheral arterial disease causes loss of sensitivity in the lower extremities which is why it is not recommended to apply direct heat to the affected limbs as it puts the client at great risk for burning.

Elevating the legs, no higher than the level of the heart, joining a prescribed exercise program, and regular inspection of skin integrity and the affected limbs in general are all appropriate actions for the condition.

53.

Answer- A

Explanation: The side effects of taking lovastatin are:

-Headache, dizziness, blurring of vision
- Gastric disturbances: nausea, either diarrhea or constipation, flatulence
-Abdominal cramps, muscle cramps
-Fatigue
-Raised liver enzyme levels
-Pruritis, skin rash

54.

Answer- A

Explanation: The primary description of Reynaud's disease is the presence of vasospasms to the blood vessels of both the upper and lower limbs. Vasodilators are prescribed to manage this.

55.

Answer- B

Explanation: Recovery for myocarditis is usually spontaneously even without medical intervention.

56.

Answer- B

Explanation: Too much feeling of anxiety can overpower the analgesic effect of pain medication for angina. Learning relaxation techniques or methods to reduce stress and anxiety can help to elevate a client's response to the medication.

57.

Answer- B

Explanation: Raised levels of creatinine phosphokinase (CPK) are often seen in injuries involving the muscles. CPK MB's are elevated when damage to the myocardium happens.

58.

Answer- A

Explanation: Beta-adrenergic blockers, such as sotalol, is contraindicated for clients with asthma, therefore a change of drug must be discussed. Checking the blood pressure and apical pulse of the client prior to administration are also relevant but not the foremost priority in this situation.

59.

Answer- A

Explanation: Part of the preoperative teaching is to inform the client that an endotracheal tube will be inserted and the client will be put on a mechanical ventilator.

60.

Answer- A

Explanation: When a client is on both antilipemic therapy and anticoagulant therapy, the dosage for the anticoagulant should be decreased as the two medications compete with one another.

61.

Answer- D

Explanation: A premature ventricular contraction every other heartbeat is called bigeminy. Trigeminy is a PVC every third heartbeat while quadrigeminy is a PVC every fourth heartbeat. A couplet or pair is two sequential premature ventricular contractions.

62.

Answer- A

Explanation: An effective pericardiocentesis is characterized by a decreased central venous pressure. The other options are expected outcomes of a successful procedure.

63.

Answer- B

Explanation: The client's permanent pacemaker may be deactivated by the highly magnetic fields used for imaging.

64.

Answer- A

Explanation: Keeping the oxygen turned on during the procedure is a fire hazard. All the other options are proper precautions taken when performing cardioversion.

65.

Answer- C

Explanation: Adrenergic agonists stimulate the beta receptors to increase both the cardiac output and the myocardial force in clients with heart failure or who are undergoing cardiopulmonary bypass surgery. The side effects of this medication are:
- Angina
- Urinary urgency or incontinence
- Tachycardia
- Restlessness
- Dysrhythmias

66.

Answer- A

Explanation: The pain described by the client is typical of Prinzmetal's or variant angina. Stable angina is precipitated by physical activity or exercise and is relieved by rest and medication. Unstable angina is not as predictable and most often leads to myocardial infarction.

67.

Answer- B

Explanation: Dizziness is one of the signs of procainamide toxicity but it can also be caused by several other conditions. Before any intervention can be carried out, a client assessment should be done first.

68.
Answer- B

Explanation: A sclerosing agent, hence the term sclerotherapy, is injected into the varicose vein. This agent causes damage to the venous walls which in turn closes the vein and disrupts local blood flow. The surgical removal of varicose veins is called vein ligation and stripping where the vein is tied off and removed with a hook.

69.

Answer- A

Explanation: It is recommended to maintain a semi-Fowler's position as one of the postoperative nursing interventions following placement of a vena caval filter.

70.

Answer- A

Explanation: The normal digoxin levels are from 0.5 ng/mg to 2.0 ng/mg. A laboratory value beyond the upper limit of that range would most likely lead to digoxin toxicity.

71.

Answer- B

Explanation: The presenting signs and symptoms of the client are all indicative of heart failure.

72.

Answer- C

Explanation: The maximum number of sublingual nitroglycerin tablets to be taken is three: one every five minutes. If the pain is persistent and is not relieved after taking a total of three tablets then the physician must be informed immediately.

73.

Answer- A

Explanation: The apical pulse is auscultated at the approximate location of the heart's apex (maximum point of impulse) which is generally located at the fourth to fifth intercostals space at the midclavicular line.

74.

Answer- A

Explanation: Hypertensive clients are advised to read food labels and nutritional information labels to determine the sodium levels of consumable items. For the options presented, demineralized water has the lowest sodium level among all the choices.

75.

Answer- D

Explanation: Checking the label of the lidocaine vial for its components or additives ensures that the nurse does not administer a preparation meant as a local anesthetic. Lidocaine used as local anesthesia contains epinephrine and/ or a preservative.

The expiration date and generic drug name are two other important things to check on any medication vial.

The color is observed by looking at the medication itself and not the label.

76.

Answer- D

Explanation: The client is most likely experiencing an anaphylactic reaction to streptokinase. The most appropriate action would be to stop the administration and refer to a physician for further management. The next step could be administration of antihistamines or corticosteroids to treat the allergic reaction.

77.

Answer- A

Explanation: The main goal of aortic aneurysm treatment is to limit or slow down the rate of the disease's progression. This is done through addressing modifiable risk factors by changing unhealthy client habits, controlling the client's blood pressure to avoid strain on the aneurysm, and initiating measures to prevent eventual rupture.

78.

Answer- C

Explanation: The client's complaints are side effects caused by nitrates. It is important to inform the client on what to expect after medication usage. If the side effects are intolerable to the client, the nurse may refer the case to a physician for readjustment of dosage or drug substitution.

79.

Answer- D

Explanation: An expected side effect of nicotinic acid is flushing. Taking a non-steroidal anti-inflammatory drug (NSAID) can decrease this occurrence.

80.

Answer- A

Explanation: Excessive straining especially during a bowel movement may precipitate an angina episode. Other triggering situations include:

-   Strenuous physical activity
-   Smoking
-   Emotional stress
-   Extreme heat or cold

81.

Answer- B

Explanation: Furosemide (Lasix) is a loop diuretic diuretic that may cause the excretion of water, electrolytes, and calcium. This may put the client at risk for developing hypokalemia.

All the other options are potassium-sparing diuretics that promote retention of potassium which would put the clients at risk for hyperkalemia

82.

Answer- A

Explanation: Using an electrocardiogram is the fastest and easiest way to determine the location of myocardial damage.

Cardiac Enzymes are included in the diagnostics involved with myocardial infarction but cannot be used to determine the location

Cardiac catheterization may also be employed to determine the location of damage but it us usually not performed immediately as the first diagnostic tool choice.

83.

Answer- B

Explanation: Assessing the patient is the nurse's priority in this situation to identify what is the most appropriate course of action to take next. Initiating CPR or referring to a physician may be done after assessment

depending on the findings.
84.

Answer- A

Explanation: A third degree atrioventricular heart block is also referred to as Mobitz II. On the other hand, a second-degree atrioventricular heart block is sometimes called as Mobitz I.

85.

Answer- B

Explanation: The unclear ECG tracing might be caused by several factors such as:
-Incorrect lead placement
-Loose cables and wires
-Excessive patient movement
-Placing the leads on a hairy surface

86.

Answer- C

Explanation: Protamine sulfate is the antidote for heparin.
Vitamin K is the antidote for warfarin (Coumadin), another anticoagulant.

87.

Answer- A

Explanation: All the options are important however oxygenation and relieving the client's pain are the first priorities in the initial treatment of acute myocardial infarction (MI).

88.

Answer- D

Explanation: Pain caused by a pulmonary condition becomes worse upon inhaling.

All the other options are questions asked as a part of the standard pain assessment but may or may not be helpful in determining the origin or cause of the chest pain.

89.

Answer- B

Explanation: Ethacrynic acid is a loop diuretic, urea is an osmotic diuretic, methazolamide is a carbonic anhydrase inhibitor, and amiloride is a potassium-sparing diuretic.

90.

Answer- B

Explanation: It is best to take the blood pressure of a

client after being rested for thirty minutes after smoking or consuming caffeinated beverages. All the other choices are examples of good nursing practice and should be encouraged instead of avoided.

91.

Answer- A

Explanation: Resuscitative equipment should be prepared in case of any untoward incident. Other appropriate interventions are:
-Connecting the client to a cardiac monitor
-Obtaining an ECG tracing before, during, and after the procedure
-Continuous monitoring of cardiac rhythm

Emptying the bladder and specimen collection is not an immediate concern for the procedure.

A carotid sinus massage involves turning the clients head to the side.

92.

Answer- B

Explanation: A heart attack is a general nonmedical term used to describe the condition where there is damage to the cardiac muscles caused by reduced blood flow to the heart. The root cause may be myocardial infarction or coronary artery disease.

Brain attack is sometimes used to refer to a stroke.

Stroke is caused by reduced blood flow to the brain.

Syncope is sometimes interchanged with fainting and is defined as a temporary unconsciousness usually associated with reduced blood flow to the brain.

93.

Answer- D

Explanation: Non-steroidal anti-inflammatory drugs (NSAIDs) such as aspirin can cause damage to the gastric linings which would in turn exacerbate the client's peptic ulcers.

94.

Answer- B

Explanation: Antihistamines and corticosteroids may be administered to a client who is allergic to any of the components of the radiopaque dye used for angiography. This prevents any anaphylactic reactions and allows for the completion of the procedure.

95.

Answer- A

Explanation: Hypersensitivity, a tingling sensation, or a feeling of being poked by numerous needles may be an indication of injury to the saphenous nerve. This finding should be made known to a physician.

96.

Answer- C

Explanation: Defibrillation can be done up to a maximum of three times, with the fist shock at the lowest energy level of 200 Joules moving up to 300 Joules and 360 Joules for the subsequent shocks.

97.

Answer- A

Explanation: Ventricular tachycardia lowers the cardiac output which leads to ischemia in the heart and brain tissues.

98.

Answer- B

Explanation: Thrombophlebitis can escalate to pulmonary embolism if the thrombus has been dislodged and travels to the respiratory area. The signs and symptoms of pulmonary embolism include:

- Sudden chest pain
- Cough
- Shortness of breath
- Anxiety
- Excessive sweating or diaphoresis

99.

Answer- C

Explanation: The most common complication after the insertion of pacemakers is the dislodgment of the device's pacing electrode. Limiting arm movements on the affected side will decrease the possibility of dislodgment.

100.

Answer- B

Explanation: Cardiopulmonary resuscitation (CPR) is indicated for asystole. Other interventions to treat asystole include administration of adrenaline and/ or epinephrine.

Defibrillation is applicable only for ventricular fibrillation or pulseless ventricular tachycardia.

Lidocaine is administered as treatment for ventricular arrhythmias.

101.

Answer- A

Explanation: It is recommended for clients with a Holter monitor to avoid using bathtubs and showers as they may interfere with the device's functioning.

The Holter monitor is meant to record the client's electrocardiographic wave patterns continuously for twenty-four hours or more as he or she performs activities of daily living.

102.

Answer- C

Explanation: An echocardiogram is a noninvasive diagnostic procedure that is based on the general principles of ultrasonography. The client is positioned on his or her back and advised to avoid speaking during the test.

103.

Answer- A

Explanation: Bioprosthetic valves are grafted from animals and humans alike. Bovine valves are from cows, porcine valves are from pigs, and homografts are from human cadavers.

104.

Answer- A

Explanation: Thrombolytics are contraindicated for clients with a history of stroke.

105.

Answer- C

Explanation: Dressler's syndrome is a complication of myocardial infarction and is a combination of: pericarditis, pleural and pericardial effusion.

www.ingramcontent.com/pod-product-compliance
Lightning Source LLC
Chambersburg PA
CBHW071310220526
45468CB00001B/325